Price Comparisons for Pharmaceuticals

T0273240

Price Comparisons for Pharmaceuticals

A Review of U.S. and Cross-National Studies

Patricia M. Danzon

The AEI Press

Publisher for the American Enterprise Institute

WASHINGTON, D.C.

1999

ISBN 0-8447-7133-3

1 3 5 7 9 10 8 6 4 2

THE AEI PRESS
Publisher for the American Enterprise Institute
1150 Seventeenth Street, N.W.
Washington, D.C. 20036

Contents

1

Introduction

Several recent studies have had as their purpose "to determine whether pharmaceutical manufacturers are taking advantage of older Americans through price discrimination and, if so, whether this is part of the explanation for the high drug prices being paid by older Americans."[1] The domestic variant of these studies attempts to measure price differentials for pharmaceuticals between cash-paying customers and large health maintenance organizations in the United States. The international studies compare pharmaceutical prices paid by retail customers in the United States with those paid in Canada and Mexico.[2]

Specifically, the studies collected data for a sample of ten patented, nongeneric drugs with the highest annual sales to seniors in 1997 under the Pennsylvania Pharmaceutical Assistance Contract for the Elderly (PACE). In the domestic study (Minority Staff Domestic Report 1998a), retail pharmacy prices to cash-paying customers for the ten drugs were compared with Federal Supply Schedule (FSS) prices. The FSS is a price catalog for purchases by federal agencies. The FSS prices are interpreted as prices to "most-favored customers, such as large insurance companies and HMOs." A retail-to-FSS comparison has been done for more than twenty congressional districts. The study reviewed here looked at retail prices for the ten drugs from a sample of seventy-five pharmacies—forty-six independent and twenty-nine chain stores—in seven congressional districts. For the international comparisons, prices for the same ten drugs in retail pharmacies in a particular state or congressional district in the United States were compared with retail prices in Canada and Mexico. The study for Maine is discussed here (Minority Staff International Report 1998b).

The Domestic Report concluded that for these ten leading drugs, the average differential between the retail price to cash-paying customers and the FSS price was 106 percent. The average price differential for other, non-pharmaceutical items sold in pharmacies was only 22 percent. These differentials were attributed primarily to manufacturers' pricing policies, not to the drugstores.

The International Report concluded that the average prices in Maine to customers who buy their own drugs are 72 percent higher than the average prices in Canada and 102 percent higher than the average prices in Mexico. Both the domestic and the international reports conclude that discounts to preferred customers in the United States or abroad result in cost-shifting to U.S. retail customers, including older Americans.

The purpose of this study is to review two examples of these Minority Staff Reports, one domestic and one international. All the reports use similar methods and reach similar conclusions, and hence this study applies to them all. My main conclusion is that the Minority Staff Reports are based on flawed methodology that leads to seriously upward-biased estimates of the price differences between sectors within the United States and between the United States and Canada or Mexico. Both reports are based on a small, unrepresentative sample of five to ten branded drugs, excluding all generics. The selected drugs are all mature drugs that are expected to give disproportionately large discounts.

The reports used methods that ignore standard principles of price indexes and lead to unreliable results. The domestic study is further biased by comparing prices at different stages of the distribution chain. It compares *retail* prices (prices charged by pharmacies) to cash-paying customers with *ex-manufacturer* prices (prices charged by manufacturers) to federal customers—an "apples-to-oranges" comparison. Retail prices reflect markups charged by retail pharmacies and wholesalers, in addition to manufacturer prices, whereas the FSS price is a manufacturer-level price. The resulting estimates of the magnitude of the price differences both within the United States and between the United States and Canada or Mexico are seriously upward-biased. The reports also ignore the 24 percent mandatory discount that manufacturers of innovator drugs are required to give to the four largest federal customers.

These two omitted factors—distribution margins and statutorily required, 24 percent discounts—account for a retail-to-FSS differential of at least 65 percent, which is three-fourths of the median retail-to-FSS differential in the Minority Staff sample (86.5 percent). The reports ignore evidence from two studies based on much larger samples—GAO (1994b) and CBO (1996)—that show median best price discounts of 14–15 percent, and weighted average best price discounts of roughly 19 percent. This provides further evidence that their 106 percent differential is upward biased and atypical. And the reports focus on pharmaceuticals, ignoring the fact that discounting is common for all medical services sold to managed care and is also common in other industries. The reports also ignore the competitive benefits to consumers from discounting.

Chapter 2 of this study summarizes the standard principles for measuring price differences for pharmaceuticals. Chapter 3 reviews the domestic retail-to-FSS comparison (Minority Staff Report 1998a). Chapter 4 reviews the comparison of U.S. prices with prices in Canada and Mexico (Minority Staff Report 1998b). Chapter 5 discusses the economic basis for discounting in health care in general and pharmaceuticals in particular, including the cost-shifting argument. Chapter 6 comments briefly on the policy implications. It concludes that outpatient drug coverage for seniors is better addressed by private-sector plans, such as Medicare + Choice, than by requiring manufacturers to give FSS discounts to the retail sector. The latter strategy is expected to result in higher manufacturer prices to managed care and federal programs, with no guarantee of lower retail prices to seniors.

2

General Principles for Measuring Price Differences for Pharmaceuticals

The Minority Staff Reports violate basic principles for performing price comparisons. The comparison of prices between different markets, different countries, or different time periods poses methodological challenges that have been addressed in an extensive economic literature on price indexes.[3] Certain widely accepted principles for price comparisons are applied by the U.S. Bureau of Labor Statistics in its calculation of price indexes, and by the analogous statistical agencies in most other countries.

Sample Selection

To draw valid conclusions about the average price level for drugs to consumers in different markets, the sample must include a representative market basket of the drugs consumed. This can be achieved by taking a random sample or a stratified random sample. When the comparison is between two quite different markets—say, the United States and Mexico—the sample should be representative of both markets under comparison.

Life Cycle. In the case of pharmaceuticals, it is important to draw products from all stages of their product life, since prices can vary significantly over the life of a product and this life-cycle price profile differs across countries. For example, Berndt et al. (1993) found that the U.S. producer price index (PPI) for drugs was significantly upward-biased because of a disproportionate representation of drugs in the middle years of their life cycle and an underrepresentation of new products and generics. The sample should also be representative of the mixture of dosage forms, strengths, and packs for the products included, since the mixture of forms and packs differs significantly across countries, a reflection of regulatory, medical, and cultural differences.

Generics. A further requirement for a representative sample of pharmaceuticals is that it should include generics as well as branded originator compounds. Generics accounted for 46 percent of prescriptions in the United States in 1998, whereas generic penetration is lower in many other countries.[4] Since generics offer consumers a lower-price alternative to branded products, the exclusion of generics biases upward the estimate of the average price level in a country with relatively high generic penetration and relatively low generic prices, such as the United States. A similar logic argues for including over-the-counter (OTC) drugs, which do not require a doctor's prescription, when these offer a substitute for prescription products. Since both the market share and the relative prices of generic and OTC products differ systematically across countries in ways that are related to the regulatory regime, valid conclusions about the effects of regulation on prices must be based on samples that include generics and OTCs.

Sample-Selection Bias in the Minority Staff Reports. The Minority Staff Reports are based on a sample comprising the ten patented, nongeneric drugs with the largest annual sales to older Americans in 1997, as reported by the Pennsylvania Pharmaceutical Assistance Contract for the Elderly (PACE). PACE is a prescription drug assistance program for low-income seniors in Pennsylvania. It has a formulary of covered drugs, which are presumably selected based in part on the size of the rebate offered to PACE by manufacturers.

This sample selection violates principles of random selection and is likely to be systematically biased for several reasons. First, by focusing on leading products sold under a formulary such as PACE, the sample is likely to consist disproportionately of mature products that tend to give relatively large discounts. Simple economics predicts that, to get on formulary, manufacturers would give larger discounts, particularly to a large formulary, for mature products that have several close competitors and are nearing the end of their patent life than for newer products. The Congressional Budget Office (CBO) (1996) provides some evidence consistent with that. The conjecture that the sample is biased toward products that give relatively large discounts is supported by the evidence below. To the extent that the sample is biased toward products that give atypically large discounts, the estimates of retail-to-Federal Supply Schedule (FSS) price differentials for the sample overstate typical differentials, because large discounts to nonfederal purchasers such as PACE lead to lower FSS prices, as described below.

Second, the selection criterion admits only patented drugs, even though generics account for 46 percent of prescriptions countrywide in the United States. Third, since the selection criterion is products with the highest annual sales by dollar value rather than by number of prescriptions, the sample is biased toward products with relatively high prices, other factors being equal.

Matching Drugs across Markets

Ideally, prices should be compared for products that are identical in all relevant respects in the different markets—

the same active ingredient, same manufacturer, same brand name, same dosage form, same strength, same pack size. In practice, a given compound is often produced by different manufacturers in different countries, because of licensing and generic entry; and most products are available in several dosage forms, strengths, and pack sizes, which also differ across countries. Given this heterogeneity in the product range, applying strict matching criteria excludes many products from the comparison and hence makes it unrepresentative. Thus, there is a trade-off. If strict comparability is required along all possible dimensions (chemical composition, manufacturer, dosage form, strength, pack size), the sample of drugs that can be included in the comparison will be a very small and nonrepresentative subset of the range of medicines that is available to consumers in each country. In particular, the requirement of matching the manufacturer or brand is counterproductive, because it limits the comparison to compounds sold internationally by subsidiaries of multinational companies—and automatically excludes most generics and licensed products.

The preferred approach is therefore to compare the price of the molecule, computed as the volume-weighted average of prices charged by all manufacturers of the compound, including the originator, licensees, and generic manufacturers (Danzon and Kim 1998). This implicitly assumes that generics are perfect substitutes for the innovator brand. Although the assumption may be too strong in some cases, it is less misleading than the assumption that generics are not substitutes, which is implied by omitting generics from the comparison, as the Minority Staff have done. Indeed, treating generics as perfect substitutes for brands is consistent with the reimbursement practices of most managed pharmacy benefit programs and Medicaid in the United States, and with public payers in Canada, Germany, and the United Kingdom.

Retail versus Wholesale versus Manufacturer Price

In principle, prices for pharmaceuticals can be measured at three points on the distribution chain: the ex-manufacturer price is the price at which the manufacturer sells to the wholesaler; the ex-wholesale price is the price at which the wholesaler sells to the retail pharmacy; and the retail price is the price at which the pharmacy sells to the consumer. Thus, the retail price differs from the ex-manufacturer price because of the wholesale and retail distribution markups. Value-added taxes further widen the gap in some countries. In practice, true transactions prices may not be readily observable because of discounts related to volume, cash payment, and such, and because the manufacturer prices and the wholesale and retail markups may differ by class of customer, product, and location.

In general, because retail prices include significant distribution markups that differ across markets and between products within some markets, comparisons of retail prices do not provide accurate measures of differences in ex-manufacturer prices. To make comparisons at retail-price levels, as the Minority Staff International Report purports to do, information on the wholesale and retail margins is also required if these retail-price comparisons are to serve as a basis for valid inferences about differences in ex-manufacturer prices.

The Minority Staff Domestic Report is an apples-to-oranges comparison, because it compares retail prices to cash customers with the FSS price, which is an ex-manufacturer price. I discuss the matter in detail in chapter 3, below.

Price and Volume Measures

There are several possible measures of quantity for pharmaceuticals, each with a corresponding measure of price—

for example, price per pack, price per pill or dose, price per daily dose, price per course of therapy, or price per gram of active ingredient. Because countries differ in their range of dosage forms, pack sizes, strengths, and such, comparisons are sensitive to the unit of measure used (see Danzon and Kim 1998).

Moreover, a comparison that is based on price for a single strength or dosage form, or for a pack size that is "common" in the United States, does not provide an accurate measure of price per course of therapy on average in the United States or in the comparison countries. That is because the price per pill and the price per pack vary with pack size within and across countries. In particular, price per pill tends to decrease as pack size increases, and price per gram tends to decrease with average strength. Some countries, including the United States and Canada, permit distribution in very large packs to pharmacists who then split the packs for retail distribution. Other countries, which do not permit pharmacists to split packs, have much smaller average pack sizes, which leads to a higher price per pill, since the price per pill is typically lower in larger packs.

The Minority Staff Reports compare prices for a single strength of a single form (tablets) and pack size that is supposedly typical for the United States. The largest U.S. packs, which have the lowest price per pill, were apparently not used in the studies. For drugs that were included in the 1992 GAO comparison of prices in the United States and Canada, the reports used the same pack; for drugs not included in the 1992 GAO study, they used the "dosage, form, and package size common in the years 1994 through 1997." The reports give no information about how a price was estimated for the comparison countries if comparable packs were not available or were atypical. The 1992 GAO study used a larger pack size in Canada than in the United States, which contributed to the upward-biased estimates of U.S.-Canadian price differentials in that study. A similar bias probably applies to the Minority Staff Reports (1998a, b), but no information is given.

Standard Price Indexes: Weighting of Products

An accurate comparison of the cost of medicines to consumers in different markets requires weighting the prices of different products in the market basket to reflect their relative importance in overall expenditures. When the relative importance of different medicines differs considerably across countries, there is no unique "best" weighting scheme. The analyst should choose the weights most appropriate to the context and question at issue.

The economic literature on price measurement has developed several standard price indexes, each of which reflects different assumptions and results in a different measure of cross-country price differences. In the context of a bilateral international price comparison between, say, Canada and the United States as a base, the Laspeyres index weights each price by the volume of the United States.[5] The Paasche index uses Canadian weights. The Fisher index is the geometric mean of the Laspeyres and Paasche indexes. If the current policy question is, What would be the cost of medicines to U.S. consumers if they faced Canadian prices?, then a Laspeyres index that uses U.S. consumption weights is appropriate. This implicitly assumes that U.S. doctors and consumers would be unlikely to switch to Canadian consumption patterns, at least in the short run, even if faced with Canadian prices.

The Minority Staff Reports base their conclusions on the simple average of the price ratios, expressed as a percentage of the lower price, for the ten products. There is no weighting for volume differences. The unweighted average is inconsistent with basic principles of index numbers (see Diewert 1987). This simple average is extremely sensitive to the particular items in the sample. For example, in the ten-drug sample, if the two largest numbers are omitted, the average differential declines from 106 percent to 83 percent. Conversely, if the calculation includes two other drugs for which differentials of 1,407 percent and 584 percent are reported, the average differential increases from 106 percent to 254 percent! Clearly, the sample and the methods used here do not provide a robust measure of average price differences.

3

The U.S. Retail Price versus FSS Best Price Comparison

The Minority Staff Domestic Report (1998a) compares the retail pharmacy price, as a measure of price to cash-paying customers, including seniors, to the Federal Supply Schedule (FSS) price, as a measure of "best price to large insurance companies and HMOs." That comparison is inappropriate because the prices are at different levels of the distribution chain.

Retail versus Ex-Manufacturer Prices

The price to cash customers is a retail price; it reflects wholesale and retail markups on top of the manufacturer price. By contrast, the FSS price is an ex-manufacturer price.[6] The Minority Staff Report (1998a, 7) acknowledges this issue but dismisses it and argues that "pharmacies appear to have relatively small markups between the prices at which they buy prescription drugs and the prices at which they sell them." The report cites two pieces of evidence to support this conclusion: "The average retail price for the ten most common drugs was only 4 percent higher than the published national Average Wholesale Price, and only 22 percent higher than the price available directly from one large wholesaler."

In fact, distribution markups contribute significantly to the differences between retail and FSS prices. Contrary to the assertion in the reports, the average wholesale price (AWP) does not measure the average transactions price charged by wholesalers. The name is misleading. The AWP is a list price published by a pricing service. It serves as a benchmark from which pharmacy reimbursement and discounts are calculated. But actual average wholesale prices are significantly below the AWP. For example, a leading text on managed care states that managed care plans reimburse pharmacists at AWP minus 10–17 percent (Kongstvedt 1996), which reflects the fact that pharmacists can acquire products at prices substantially below AWP. Similarly, 1997 HMO reimbursement rates to network pharmacies used an average discount off AWP of 14.2 percent, with a range of 10–20 percent (Emron 1998, Managed Care Pharmacy Director CUE Program). Thus, AWP significantly overstates the price at which pharmacies can purchase drugs.

A more plausible measure of the retail markup can be obtained using the 22 percent markup over the prices charged by the single wholesaler (McKesson) sampled in the report. The differences in ex-wholesale prices charged by different wholesalers are probably small, since the wholesale sector is highly competitive. So it is plausible to assume that the 22 percent markup is representative of the average retail markup over the wholesale price. Consistent with that assumption, a study of five leading drugs in Minnesota found that retail prices were 26 percent higher than pharmacies' wholesale acquisition cost— which means that the 22 percent retail markup used here may be conservative.

In addition, to obtain the ex-manufacturer price, the wholesale margin must also be subtracted. That, typically, is about 2–4 percent of the average manufacturer's price (AMP).[7] Using these estimates of distribution margins, if the AMP is 100, then the ex-wholesale price is 103, and the retail price is 125.7 (100 x 1.03 x 1.22). Thus, retail prices overstate the ex-manufacturer prices in the retail segment by roughly 25.7 percent.

The Federal Supply Schedule

The Federal Supply Schedule for pharmaceuticals is a price catalog for purchases by federal agencies, including the Department of Veterans Affairs (VA), the Department of Defense (DOD), the Public Health Service (PHS), the Coast Guard, and the Indian Health Service. The VA is the largest single purchaser and accounts for 71 percent of purchases from the pharmaceutical FSS in fiscal year 1996 (GAO 1997). It is also responsible for negotiating the FSS prices with drug manufacturers. Under the Veterans Health Care Act of 1992 (P.L. 102-585 sec. 603), manufacturers of innovator drugs—single and multiple-source—must make their products available on the FSS if the products are to be eligible for reimbursement by Medicaid. Thus, manufacturers face a significant economic penalty for failure to participate in the FSS. This, in turn, gives the VA leverage in negotiating FSS prices.

Under General Services Administration (GSA) procurement regulations, in negotiating prices for the FSS the VA must seek a price that "represents the same discount off a drug's list price that the manufacturer offers its most-favored nonfederal customer under comparable terms and conditions" (GAO 1997, 6, citing 48 C.F.R. sec. 538.270). To determine this best price, manufacturers are required to submit a commercial sales practices (CSP) form, which provides information by product on prices, terms, and conditions set for different customers. Whether the VA considers a particular customer "comparable" may be subject to negotiation and depends on various factors, including the terms and conditions of the commercial sale.

The Veterans Health Care Act also requires manufacturers of innovator drugs to sell them to four agencies—

the VA, the DOD, the PHS, and the Indian Health Service—at a discount of at least 24 percent off their nonfederal average manufacturer price (NFAMP). An excess inflation rebate is also required, equal to the percentage by which the price increase for this drug has exceeded the consumer price index (CPI) in the prior period. Thus, the federal ceiling price (FCP) is equal to NFAMP x 0.76 x $(1 - p)$, where $p \geq 0$ is the excess inflation rebate. The NFAMP is a weighted average price for all nonfederal classes of trade, for each dosage form and strength, that wholesalers pay, net of any cash discounts and chargebacks. Thus, discounts to all private customers are reflected in the NFAMP if those discounts are given directly to wholesalers. Omitted from the NFAMP are rebates that are given directly to final purchasers, such as a rebate given to a large HMO contingent on demonstrated market-share performance. The mandatory FCP discount applies to innovator products even after patent expiration. For generic products there is no FCP.

For innovator products, the FSS price may in theory be higher or lower than the FCP, depending on whether the best price to a comparable nonfederal customer is less or greater than the mandated FCP discount. If the FSS price exceeds the FCP, however, the VA, DOD, PHS, and Indian Health Service, which account for the great majority of FSS sales, would pay only the FCP. So the FCP tends to act as a ceiling on the FSS price. Thus, the FSS price tends to be the lower of either (1) the federal ceiling price, which is NFAMP x 0.76 x $(1 - p)$, or (2) the lowest price given to a comparable nonfederal purchaser.

The evidence from a recent GAO report indicates that, for the majority of originator products, the FSS price is determined by the FCP-mandated discount. In a review of FSS prices relative to the FCP for schedule drugs as of September 30, 1996, the GAO (1997a) found that about 73 percent of products—mostly generics—were not subject to the FCP. Although those FCP-exempt products account for a large fraction of products (a "product" is a single dosage form or pack), they account roughly for only 25 percent of sales to the VA. The remaining 27 percent of products, which account for about 75 percent of sales, are subject to the FCP. These are the innovator products that are the subject of the Minority Staff Reports (1998a, b). Of these innovator products, 72 percent (or 19.3 percent of all products) had an FSS price at or above the FCP, which implies that the best price to private customers was less than the mandated FCP.[8] Only 8 percent of products (28 percent of innovator products) had an FSS price below FCP—and hence had best prices to private customers that were lower than the mandated FCP, as defined by a discount of 24 percent plus excess inflation off NFAMP.[9]

Moreover, simple economics predicts that most private discounts are no greater than the minimum Medicaid-mandated discount of 15.1 percent off AMP, because any larger discount would also have to be given to Medicaid. The Omnibus Budget Reconciliation Act of 1990 (OBRA) tried to reduce Medicaid's prescription drug costs by requiring that manufacturers give state Medicaid programs a discount equal to the greater of the following two possibilities: (1) a fixed percentage (12.5 percent in 1991–1992, 15.7 percent in 1993, 15.4 percent in 1994, 15.2 percent in 1995, and 15.1 percent thereafter) off the average manufacturer price to wholesalers for distribution to the retail class of trade, or (2) the best price given to any private customer. This matching requirement greatly increases the cost to manufacturers of giving discounts in excess of 15.1 percent to private customers. Giving a discount greater than 15.1 percent to a private customer would increase net revenue only if the additional private volume induced by the discount offset the lower price per unit on those private sales *and* the revenue that is lost because of the lower price per unit on sales to Medicaid.

Since Medicaid accounts for 11 percent of sales on average, the Medicaid volume would usually be several times larger than any incremental private volume induced by the discount and would thereby make such discounting in excess of 15.1 percent off AMP rarely worthwhile.

The evidence from the GAO (1994b) and the CBO (1996) is consistent with the prediction from simple economics that requiring manufacturers to give their best price discount to Medicaid would reduce the discounts offered to private customers to the mandatory minimum discount of 15.1 percent. In a study of the effects of OBRA 1990, the GAO (1994b) found that, between 1991 and 1993, the median best price discount given to HMOs declined from 24.4 percent to 14.2 percent. For group purchasing organizations (GPOs) the median best price discount declined from 27.8 percent to 15.3 percent.[10] Thus, by the first quarter of 1993, the median best price discount to private managed purchasers had fallen to about the minimum rebate required by OBRA, roughly 15 percent of AMP (see figure 3–1). Similarly, the CBO (1996) found that the weighted average best price in a sample of roughly 800 brand-name products declined from 36.7 percent in 1991 to 19.3 percent in 1994 (see table 3–1). Although the evidence is taken from 1993 and 1994, it is likely still to be relevant, since the Medicaid best price provisions are unchanged.

The CBO (1996) notes that best price discounts on some products may still exceed 15.1 percent for several reasons. Larger discounts are more common for products with several competitors than for recently launched, single-source products; products with relatively small sales to Medicaid; and products for certain end users, such as academic medical centers.

The evidence that median best price discounts given to private customers are roughly 15 percent of the average manufacturer price to the retail sector, and hence much

FIGURE 3–1
Changes in Median Best Price Discounts
for HMO and GPO Drugs, 1991–1993
Percentage

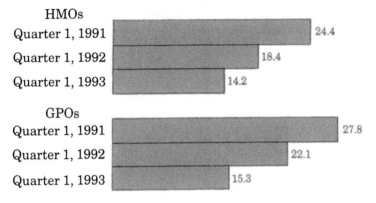

Source: U.S. General Accounting Office, "Medicaid Changes in Best Price for Outpatient Drugs Purchased by HMOs and Hospitals," August 1994.

smaller than the 106 percent average differential cited by the Minority Staff Reports, is further supported by estimates of savings achieved by pharmacy benefit management companies (PBMs). PBMs act on behalf of insurance companies, HMOs, and self-insured employers to manage the pharmacy benefit. This involves negotiating discounts on drug prices with drug manufacturers and discounts on retail pharmacy margins with pharmacies that participate in the network. In a study of the effect of PBMs done for the Federal Employee Health Benefit Program (FEHBP), the GAO (1997a) estimated that PBMs reduced total pharmacy benefit costs by 20–27 percent, relative to what those costs would have been without the PBM. Of the total savings, the share attributed to manufacturer discounts was at most 21 percent, or 4–6 percent of total pharmacy benefit costs. A much larger share (52 percent

TABLE 3–1

AVERAGE BEST PRICE DISCOUNTS, 1991–1994

(percent)

| | | All Drugs | | Top 100 Drugs, |
Year	Quarter	Weighted	Unweighted	Unweighted
1991	1	36.7	42.1	35.1
	2	35.8	41.7	34.1
	3	35.4	41.1	33.6
	4	35.0	39.5	33.2
1992	1	27.8	37.7	27.8
	2	26.7	36.7	27.8
	3	28.2	36.9	27.8
	4	24.9	33.4	24.7
1993	1	20.2	29.2	18.8
	2	20.2	28.5	18.5
	3	19.8	26.3	18.5
	4	19.9	25.7	18.8
1994	1	18.5	25.0	18.8
	2	19.3	25.2	19.3

SOURCE: U.S. Congressional Budget Office, "How the Medicaid Rebate on Prescription Drugs Affects Pricing in the Pharmaceutical Industry," January 1996.

of the savings, or 10–14 percent of total pharmacy benefit costs) was attributed to retail and mail-order pharmacy discounts. Maximum-allowable-cost (MAC) reimbursement for multisource compounds was the third largest source of savings, yielding 14 percent of the total.[11] The figures for the FEHBP are similar to the conventional wisdom on savings from PBMs. The quite modest savings are further evidence that the Minority Staff Reports' estimate of manufacturer discounts of 106 percent is grossly exaggerated as a measure of typical discounts.

There are several reasons why manufacturers may be willing, in some circumstances, to accept an FSS price that is low relative to much of their private business. First, they are required by law to offer their products on the FSS if they wish to receive reimbursement from Medicaid: the choice is between forgoing all VA, DOD, and Medicaid reimbursement or accepting the price offered for the FSS. Since Medicaid accounts for 11 percent of sales on average and the FSS sales are an additional 1–2 percent, to refuse a listing on the FSS would entail a potentially significant loss of sales for many products.[12]

Second, negotiating to resist a demand for a low FSS price is time-consuming and costly and may not be worthwhile, as long as the FSS sales on average account for only 1–2 percent of sales. If sales at FSS prices were a larger fraction of total sales, manufacturers would surely be more resistant to large discounts, a point made by several manufacturers during the debate over extending the FSS to state and local government purchasers (see GAO 1997b).

Third, many VA hospitals are affiliated with major medical centers, and the VA is an important training ground for young physicians. Roughly 47 percent of medical residents rotate through the VA/DOD each year (U.S. Medicine, Inc. 1998). Manufacturers may thus rationally accept a relatively low price to ensure widespread use of their drugs by the physicians in training, with the expectation that the doctors would continue to use the products in their future careers. The CBO (1996) argues that relatively large discounts may be given to medical schools for similar reasons.

A Minority Staff study of five leading drugs in Minnesota (Minority Staff 1999) reports a 124 percent retail-to-federal price differential.[13] For the federal price, the study used the lowest federal price available. For three of the five drugs, this was the FSS price. For one drug the lowest price was the VA formulary price, and for another it was the VA's Blanket Pricing Agreement (BPA) price. Both the VA formulary price and the BPA price are prices given in return for preferred status or volume performance. Not surprisingly, they are often lower than the FSS price.

Accounting for the Retail-to-FSS Price Differential

A simple calculation shows that the statutory 24 percent FCP discount and the retail and wholesale distribution margins account for a retail-to-FSS price differential of 65 percent. Adding in a discount of 15 percent to private customers raises the implied differential to 95 percent. To demonstrate this, recall first the calculation above showing that, if AMP is 100, retail price is 125.7. Next, make the conservative assumptions that, because of minimal discounting to private customers, the NFAMP is equal to AMP, and the FSS price is equal to the FCP price, with the mandated minimum discount of 24 percent off NFAMP. So if NFAMP = AMP = 100, FSS is 76. With those conservative estimates, the implied retail-to-FSS markup is 65.4 percent (1.257 / 0.76). Thus, the combination of statutorily required discounts and distribution markups accounts for a 65.4 percent differential between retail and FSS price (see figure 3–2).

Alternatively, if we assume an average discount to private payers of 15 percent off AMP, then NFAMP = .85 AMP, and the implied retail-to-FSS markup is 94.6 percent (1.257 / (0.76 x 0.85)). If the average private discount is 10 percent, such that NFAMP = .9 AMP, then the implied retail-to-FSS markup is 84 percent (1.257 / (0.76 x 0.9)). To the extent that FCP includes an excess inflation rebate, such that the statutory discount off NFAMP ex-

FIGURE 3–2
How Distribution Margins and Mandated Discounts Contribute to Retail-to-FSS Ratio

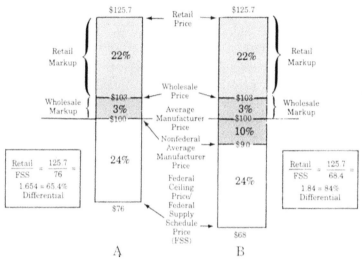

Source: Author. See text.

ceeds 24 percent, the retail-to-FSS differential attributable solely to distribution margins and legally mandated discounts would be larger. Thus, of the median retail-to-FSS differential in the Minority Staff sample of 86.5 percent, three-fourths—or 65.4 percent—can be explained solely by distribution markups and the statutorily mandated discounts. Adding an average discount to private customers of 10–15 percent would fully account for the median retail-to-FSS differential in the Minority Staff Reports (see figure 3–2).

In summary, for innovator products, manufacturers are required by law to give a federal ceiling price equal to 24 percent off the NFAMP plus any excess inflation rebate, or the best price given to a comparable customer, whichever is lower. For the majority of innovator products (72 percent in 1996), the FSS price is greater than or equal to the mandated FCP, which suggests that best prices to most favored private customers are typically above or equal to the FCP. Distribution markups and the legally mandated 24 percent FCP discounts alone imply at least a 65.4 percent retail-to-FSS differential, and more if there is an excess inflation factor. Adding a 10 percent average discount to private buyers implies an 84 percent retail-to-FSS differential. Keeping discounts to private customers at no more than 15 percent of AMP would usually be an economically rational strategy, given the Medicaid best price requirement. The evidence (GAO 1994b) confirms that the median best price discount fell to roughly 15 percent following OBRA 1990, as predicted by theory.

To the extent that the drugs in the Minority Staff Report have retail-to-FSS differentials larger than the level that can be attributed, as shown above, to distribution markups, mandated discounts, and private-sector discounts of up to 15 percent, there are at least two possible explanations. First, actual retail margins in the sample pharmacies may exceed the average estimate of 22 percent used here. Second, the drugs in the sample may be drawn disproportionately from the 28 percent of products that have discounts in excess of the mandatory minimum 24 percent FCP discount. This would be consistent with the point made earlier—that by selecting the drugs that had the largest sales under the PACE program, the Minority Staff Report sample disproportionately represents those drugs that give large discounts relative to other drugs. Thus, the evidence tends to confirm that this is not a random sample. Rather, the study appears to have sampled drugs that give atypically large discounts, and hence have atypically low FSS prices and atypically large retail-to-FSS differentials.

FSS Prices for Other Commodities

The Minority Staff Report (1998a) compares the retail-to-FSS price differential for pharmaceuticals to the price differential on a selection of other consumer items. It concludes that the average differential for the other items is only 22 percent, compared with the estimated 106 percent for pharmaceuticals.

The comparison is problematic, for several reasons. First, as noted above, manufacturers of originator drugs are required by law to give the four largest federal purchasers a discount of at least 24 percent off their average price to private purchasers. No such mandatory discount applies to other consumer products on the FSS schedule. Second, manufacturers of other products are free to choose whether or not to list their products on the FSS, with no penalty for nonparticipation other than forgoing the opportunity for sales to federal purchasers who use the schedule. By contrast, pharmaceutical manufacturers are required to list their products on the FSS as a precondition for the products' being reimbursed under the Medicaid program. Thus, the penalty for not participating, at the mandatory minimum 24 percent discount, is loss of revenue—not only from these federal purchasers but from the Medicaid program, which accounts for a much larger fraction of sales.

Third, as noted above, the retail markups are a significant fraction of the retail price for pharmaceuticals. Although I have no data on average retail markups for other consumer products, I would expect them to be lower because there is greater competition between retail outlets in supplying those other products than in supplying drugs. Moreover, the demand for drugs is likely to be more inelastic than the demand for other consumer goods, because of insurance coverage for some cash-paying customers, the essential nature of some drugs, and the fact that prescribing decisions are made by physicians, who are often uninformed or unconcerned about the relative prices of different drugs. Simple economics predicts that, if the demand for drugs is relatively inelastic, pharmacists will rationally charge higher markups on drugs than on other consumer items for which demand is more elastic.

Given the mandatory FCP discount, the greater penalty on pharmaceutical manufacturers for not participating in the FSS, and the greater distribution markups on drugs, it is not surprising that the retail-versus-FSS price differential is greater for pharmaceuticals than for other consumer products.

4

Comparisons with Canada and Mexico

The Minority Staff Report (1998b) compares prices for the same ten brand-name prescription drugs in the United States with prices at a sample of four pharmacies in three provinces of Canada and three pharmacies in one town in Mexico. The report finds that prices on average are 72 percent higher in Maine than in Canada and 102 percent higher than in Mexico. It concludes that "drug manufacturers appear to be engaged in 'cost-shifting.' They charge low prices to consumers in Canada and Mexico and appear to make up the difference by charging far higher prices to senior citizens and other individual consumers in the United States."

There are several reasons why drug prices may be lower in Canada and Mexico. However, this study is based on severely flawed methodology and seriously overestimates the actual average differences.

Canada

Several factors may contribute to lower drug prices in Canada. First, there is lower exposure to product liability in Canada. Manning (1997) finds that liability is a significant factor contributing to higher prices in the United States than in Canada. Second, Canada's federal government controls the prices of new products, and post-launch price increases are not permitted to exceed the rate of increase of the consumer price index (CPI). Third, until recently, these price controls operated under threat of compulsory licensing. If a manufacturer did not accept the government's price, the government could force the manufacturer of a patented product to license a generic producer to manufacture the product, even though that nullified the patent protection. Under the North American Free Trade Agreement (NAFTA), this compulsory licensing is no longer permitted. But the prices of products that were on the market under the compulsory licensing regime could still be affected, because restrictions on price increases would prevent a catch-up price increase. Fourth, in addition to the federal government's controls, some provincial governments in Canada operate other control mechanisms, such as the reference-price system in British Columbia, which may constrain prices below the price permitted by the federal controls. Fifth, retail distribution markups may be lower in Canada than in the cash sector in the United States. Precise comparisons are not possible because retail markups in Canada differ by province and by product.

Although these factors could lead to somewhat lower prices in Canada than in the United States, the Minority Staff Report's conclusion that "the average prices that senior citizens [in the United States] must pay are 72 percent higher than the average prices that Canadian consumers must pay" is exaggerated because the methodology of the study is flawed. First, it is based on a sample of only ten products, all brand-name products that are leaders by dollar volume of U.S. sales, and hence selected to be relatively high-priced, other things being equal. The sample excludes all generics, although generics account for more than 46 percent of prescriptions in the United States and are priced relatively low. The sample also excludes over-the-counter (OTC) products.

Second, the study generally used the same single dosage, form, and package size—when they were available—as were used by the 1992 GAO report comparing prices in the United States and Canada. For the latter study, when the U.S. price was for a pack of 100 but that pack was not available in Canada, the GAO set a Canadian price by linear imputation. For example, the price for a pack of 100 tablets was imputed by dividing the Ontario government's price for a pack of 1,000 tablets by 10. Since price per tablet is typically lower in larger packs, the methodology results in systematic downward bias in estimates of Canadian prices relative to the United States. No information is given on the selection of pack size for Mexico, but if the same linear imputation is used, then similar bias is likely. Moreover, the same linear imputations were apparently made for strength, which could further bias the estimates of U.S./Mexican differentials.

Third, the ten drugs are weighted equally, ignoring differences in market shares. As noted in chapter 2, these sample-selection and weighting procedures are not robust and violate basic principles of price indexes that are accepted and used not only by academics but also by the Bureau of Labor Statistics and similar statistical agencies in other countries. For example, since the differentials for individual products range from 23 percent to 136 percent, the overall average is very sensitive to adding or deleting individual drugs from the sample.

The Minority Staff Report states that its finding, that retail prices are 72 percent higher in the United States than in Canada, "is broadly consistent with the findings of other analysis. In 1992, the General Accounting Office looked at the prices that drug companies charge wholesalers for 121 prescription drugs and found that these prices were, on average, 32 percent higher in the United States than in Canada." Since the 1992 study was of ex-manufacturer prices and the 1998 study was of retail prices, if both purport to describe the same market differentials as the Minority Staff Report claims, this would imply that retail pharmacy markups add an additional 40 percentage points in the United States as compared with Canada! The report does not comment on this implication. It also does not comment on the fact that its 72 percent estimate of the differential is 125 percent higher than the GAO estimate of 32 percent, contrary to its claim that the findings are "broadly consistent." In fact, the differences between these two estimates are not surprising. They further illustrate the sensitivity of comparisons to small and unrepresentative samples, particularly when the comparison is based on an unweighted average, as was used in both the 1998 Minority Staff Report and the 1992 GAO report.[14]

To provide more reliable estimates of international price differences, we constructed price indexes using standard index-number methods applied to fully comprehensive data on all drugs available in the United States, Canada, and several other major markets in 1992. Using U.S. consumption patterns as the weights and comparing price per dose, our estimates of foreign prices relative to the United States are as follows: Canada +3.0 percent; Germany +27.3 percent; France –29.9 percent; Italy –9.3 percent; Japan –7.7 percent; Switzerland +44.4 percent; Sweden +8.9 percent; and the United Kingdom –23.9 percent (see table 4–1).[15] Note that these comparisons based on ex-manufacturer list prices do not reflect discounts to managed care, hospitals, and government purchasers in the United States. Thus, these comparisons overstate average manufacturer prices in the United States relative to the comparison countries.

A major conclusion of our analysis is that measures of international price differences for pharmaceuticals are very sensitive to the unit for measuring price, sample, and weights used. We computed the comparisons using price

TABLE 4-1
PRICE COMPARISONS FOR ALL MATCHING
SINGLE-MOLECULE DRUGS, 1992
(U.S. weights)

	Price/Gram	Price/Dose	Number of Molecules
Canada	−13.0	+3.0	458
Germany	−2.8	+27.3	471
France	−43.0	−29.9	412
Italy	−26.1	−9.3	406
Japan	+28.2	−7.7	396
Switzerland	+4.9	+44.4	308
Sweden	−18.9	+8.9	261
United Kingdom	−32.2	−23.9	453

Source: Danzon, Patricia M. "The Uses and Abuses of International Price Comparisons," in *Competitive Strategies in the Pharmaceutical Industry,* edited by Robert B. Helms (Washington, D.C.: AEI Press, 1996).

per gram as well as price per dose, using different samples and different weighting schemes. For example, for Japan the estimates range from 28.2 percent higher than for the United States, using price per gram and U.S. weights, to 55.2 percent lower than for the United States, using price per dose and Japanese consumption weights. There is no single "right" number. These estimates based on the full sample of products and packs and using standard index number methods, however, are clearly more accurate than the GAO estimate, which was based on an unweighted average of prices for 121 drugs, using a single pack per drug and omitting all generics. It is noteworthy that using this distorted sample and inappropriate methods, GAO (1992) estimated the United States as 32 percent higher than Canada (or Canada as 24 percent lower than the United States). Using our fully representative sample, however, along with appropriate methods and U.S. consumption weights, Canada was shown to be 3 percent higher than the United States based on price per dose, and 13 percent lower based on price per gram (Danzon 1996; Danzon and Kim 1998; see also table 4–1).

Mexico

Mexico is not an appropriate benchmark for price comparisons with the United States for several reasons. Mexico is at a less advanced stage of economic development, has lower real wages and per capita incomes, and has lower prices for many goods and services. A recent study, *The Health Care System in Mexico* (NERA 1998), reports Mexican average per capita gross national product (GNP) at U.S.$3,670 in 1996, using market exchange rates (U.S.$7,660 using purchasing power parity (PPP) exchange rates, which take into account differences in price levels between countries). Per capita expenditure on health care is estimated at 4.7 percent of gross domestic product (GDP) in 1997, or less than half the percentage spent by the United States (13.5) from its much higher per capita GDP (Anderson and Poulier 1999). Per capita spending on health care was $391 in 1997 in Mexico, compared with $3,925 in the United States. Medicines accounted for 28–32 percent of total health care spending (NERA 1998), a higher percentage than in most Organization for Economic Cooperation and Development (OECD) countries, although comparable to other less developed countries. By comparison, in 1995 the proportion of health expenditure devoted to pharmaceuticals was 8.5 percent in the United States; 13.6 percent in Canada; 15.9 percent in the United Kingdom; and 16.7 percent in France (NERA 1998, 77).

The National Economic Research Associates (NERA) study points out that the range of pharmaceuticals is very different in Mexico than in the United States and other developed countries. Anti-infectives ranked first by value in Mexico, whereas they are about the fourth group in most developed countries. Cardiovasculars, which in 1996 were the top-selling group in developed countries, ranked only fifth in Mexico.

NERA reached the following conclusion on prices for pharmaceuticals in Mexico:

> The construction of indices which allow accurate comparisons of pharmaceutical prices in different countries is a difficult task. However, it appears that prices in the private sector in Mexico are lower than in most OECD countries and some support for this view can be shown by a simple comparison of average pack prices in Mexico and other countries. . . . Expressed in U.S. dollars, even in 1995, Mexican prices were less than half European prices in 1993, although the limits to the usefulness of such a calculation (e.g. it may be comparing the prices of different products or packages) should be acknowledged. [NERA 1998, 84]

NERA correctly emphasizes that conclusions based on this price comparison are tentative because it does not standardize for product mix. Nevertheless, it does strongly suggest that Mexican prices are low relative to a broad average of European prices, not just relative to U.S. prices.

I would expect several factors to contribute to these lower prices in Mexico. First, as noted above, average per capita income and average spending on health care are much lower in Mexico than in the United States. Second, Mexico did not enact patent protection for pharmaceuticals until the *Ley de Patentes* of 1991. This law did not apply patent protection to originator products already on the market, however, and did not provide for pipeline protection. Thus drugs registered prior to the legislation remain subject to competition from copy products. Copy products are products whose production could be prevented under the 1991 law, had it been in effect. Copy products are thus distinct from generics, which are legal copies introduced after patent expiration. According to NERA, "Copy products are mainly a threat for the private sector: it is estimated that 95 percent of the private market is made up of products that could potentially be copied." The potential or actual existence of cheap copy products, which do not incur the costs of research and development and information dissemination borne by originator products, makes demand for originator products more price-elastic, which constrains the prices that originator firms would rationally charge.

Third, although medicines are designated as either prescription or nonprescription (OTC) in Mexico, NERA reports that "many prescription medicines are thought, in practice, to be widely available without prescription." If so, price-sensitive consumers can more directly influence the choice between drugs than in a system such as that in the United States, where the choice between prescription products is made primarily by physicians who may not know or be concerned about product prices. To the extent that this direct consumer purchase of supposedly prescription products in Mexico is significant, it would be another factor making demand in the private market in Mexico more price-elastic than in the cash-paying market in the United States. Consistent with this, anecdotal evidence suggests that retail pharmacists in Mexico compete by offering products at prices below the minimum government price stamped on the box.

Given the lower income, government use of monopsony power, weaker patent protection, and more price-sensitive consumers in Mexico, it is not surprising that prices are lower. But since the differentials range from 20 percent to 280 percent (or more than 1,000 percent if one other product is included), this small, unrepresentative, and unweighted sample does not provide a basis for conclusions on average U.S./Mexico price differentials.

5
The Growth of Price Discounting in Health Care

I n recent years, insurance coverage of medical care, including outpatient pharmaceuticals, has undergone major changes in response to the demand for control of costs. In pharmaceuticals, managed pharmaceutical benefits are replacing the old world of unmanaged prescribing by physicians, in which patient copayments were the main constraint on spending. Indeed, the management of pharmacy benefits has spread more broadly than has managed care for other health services, as the pharmacy benefit is often carved out and managed even within traditional fee-for-service health plans.

Discounting and Managed Care

A managed pharmaceutical care strategy is an efficient response of competitive markets to the fundamental problem of health insurance. The purpose of insurance is to protect consumers from the financial burden of medical expense. But by insulating patients from costs, traditional insurance has the unfortunate effect of making consumers and providers insensitive to costs. Unrestricted insurance thus tends to encourage overuse of medical services, driving up health spending. The inevitable increase in insurance premiums is paid initially by employers and governments, but ultimately these costs must be passed on to employees, consumers, and taxpayers.

In response to the demand from consumers and payers for control over rising health-insurance premiums, insurers compete by developing strategies that control costs in ways that are least burdensome to patients. Under traditional indemnity insurance, patients and providers had virtually unlimited freedom of choice, while insurance passively paid the bill. The only constraint was patient copayment, which is a useful but limited cost control strategy. Copayments operate by reducing the patient's financial protection. But since financial protection is the reason why consumers buy insurance, copayment reduces the value of the insurance product.

The key characteristic of managed care is the use of strategies other than copayment to control costs. With managed care, insurance is no longer a passive payment mechanism. Managed care entities are actively involved in determining the type and terms of services eligible for reimbursement. Whereas traditional insurance targeted incentives to patients through copayment requirements, managed care targets the incentives of providers. A fundamental managed care strategy is to contract with selected, "cost-effective" providers who agree to accept lower prices and other contractual terms. Patients are encouraged or required to use these contract providers. Although patients thus forgo some freedom of choice, many find this less burdensome than achieving the same degree of cost restraint through copayments.

The application of managed care principles to pharmacy benefits entails the use of strategies similar to those used in managing other health services. Based on negotiations with the payer, the benefit manager establishes a formulary of preferred drugs and a network of selected retail pharmacies. Through education, financial incentives, and other strategies, physicians and patients are encouraged to use drugs on the formulary. HMOs, pharmacy benefit managers, and other entities that manage pharmaceutical benefits are able to negotiate discounted prices from manufacturers of drugs that are listed on the formulary, because on-formulary drugs tend to gain market share relative to unlisted drugs.[16] Formularies can be used to encourage generic substitution (use of a low-cost source of multisource drugs) and therapeutic interchange (substitution of a low-cost source among therapeutically similar drugs, subject to permission from the prescribing physician). Similarly, patients are encouraged to use network pharmacies that agree to accept discounted margins. The patient thus gives up some freedom of choice in return for lower cost.

The great majority of managed pharmacy benefits use formularies and generic substitution programs. Although most generic substitution programs permit members to choose brand-name over generic drugs, the patient is typically required to pay the difference or a higher copayment. Similarly, a higher copayment may be required for an off-formulary product. Thus, to compete with generics and with potential therapeutic substitutes, manufacturers of brand-name drugs must offer discounts or rebates.[17]

Patients covered by managed care plans are encouraged or required to purchase their drugs from a network of contract pharmacies or through mail order. Network pharmacies agree to accept a discounted retail margin in return for being in the network. Network participants can expect some increase in volume that is greater the more restrictive the network. Network pharmacies are generally also required to have computer capability that permits on-line checking of the patient's insurance status, monitoring drug use to ensure compliance and guard against incompatibilities, and so forth.

The strategies used for management of pharmacy

benefits are thus similar to managed care strategies for medical services in general. Network pharmacy providers and drug manufacturers agree to accept lower prices in return for the higher volume that flows to preferred providers and suppliers.

The price discounts negotiated by the pharmacy benefit manager or HMO are ultimately passed on to consumers in the form of a lower overall insurance premium, lower copayments, more comprehensive coverage, or improved convenience and service, such as on-line verification of insurance status and direct billing of the insurance plan. This pass-through of the value of discounts to consumers is sometimes questioned, and indeed it is hard to measure directly. The most telling evidence, however, is the rapid growth of the share of pharmacy benefits that are managed. The growing market share of these plans implies that consumers are willing to accept the restrictions on choice in return for the cost savings.[18] Far from being anticompetitive, price-discounting is a competitive strategy that benefits consumers.

Common Business Reasons for Price Discounting

Charging different prices to different consumers is a common business practice for many goods and services, including hospital, physician, retail pharmacy, and other medical services. There are several reasons for price discounts, including volume discounts to reflect economies of scale and quality discounts to reflect differences in service or convenience dimensions of a product or service. For example, restaurants offer early bird discounts to attract patrons at a time of day that is less convenient for most people and hence has lower opportunity cost to the restaurateur.

Perhaps most common are price discounts that may be unrelated to the manufacturer's costs but are driven by differences in the price-sensitivity of consumers. Offering a lower price to customers who are more price-sensitive is designed to increase sales to these customers, without reducing revenues from the less price-sensitive customers. For example, senior citizen discounts are commonly offered by movie theaters, buses, restaurants, and some retail pharmacies. Price-discounting of pharmaceuticals and other medical services closely resembles the discounting to price-sensitive buyers that is widely accepted in so many other markets. It would therefore be anomalous to disallow differential pricing in pharmaceuticals while permitting it for innumerable other goods and services, including other medical services. Note that a class of customers receives a discount if it is more price-sensitive than other customer classes. Age, student status, time of day, and so forth act as proxies for price sensitivity. Thus, the reason for the discounts is the same for pharmaceuticals and other services, even if the class of beneficiary is different. Seniors are targeted as price-sensitive customers for many services. But cash-paying customers, including seniors, are relatively price-insensitive customers for drugs because it is the physician, not the patient, who typically makes the product choice for drugs. Physicians tend to be price-insensitive unless they are influenced by managed care.

The Minority Staff Reports ignore the important economic distinction between discounts based on *absolute* volume, which are typically based on scale economies, and discounts based on *incremental* volume, which are motivated by price elasticity. The rationale for discounts to managed care purchasers of pharmaceuticals (and other medical services) is incremental volume, not absolute volume. Manufacturers offer discounts to HMO and pharmacy benefit managers in order for their drugs to be favored in the formulary, since formulary drugs tend to gain in market share relative to competitors. Thus discounting is a strategy to gain incremental sales and market share for the discounted drug.

By contrast, if the manufacturer were to offer discounts to one or more independent pharmacies, this might shift market share among pharmacies, if the discount is passed on as a lower price to customers, which is not guaranteed. But the discount would have no effect on the manufacturer's total volume. Total volume sold of any drug depends largely on physicians' prescribing patterns, and these are minimally affected by discounted prices to pharmacists. Any increase in volume for the manufacturer would require that patients perceive the lower price at the pharmacy and ask their physicians to switch them to the discounted drug. But most patients have little information about the relative price of alternative drugs—and may not care, if their copayment is a fixed amount per prescription, regardless of the price of the drug. Thus, if the same discount were offered by a manufacturer to retail pharmacies who sell to the cash sector, this would not have the same effect as the same discount given for incremental volume to a managed care purchaser who is thereby persuaded to give the product favored formulary status.

It has been suggested that pharmacists could influence physicians to shift their prescribing toward specific drugs, just as HMOs and other pharmacy benefit managers do. Such switching, however, would be less subject to monitoring to protect the interests of patients. A managed care formulary typically must be approved by the health plan and plan sponsor, following careful review by the pharmacy and therapeutics (P&T) committee. This review explicitly attempts to make appropriate trade-offs between lower cost to the plan and restricted choice for patients, taking into account consumer preferences as reflected in market choices among health plans. Thus, the influence that managed care formularies have over prescribing patterns is exercised subject to market pressures to ensure reasonable quality of medical care and pass-through of savings to consumers. By contrast, if a pharmacist were to induce a physician to switch to a specific drug, there is no objective review of the therapeutic merit of the switch and less assurance that the patient ultimately gets a lower price in return for switching.

Discounts Benefit Consumers

Permitting price discounting benefits consumers in two ways. Most obvious is the benefit of lower prices. Sherer (1997) suggests that permitting discounting encourages competition between drug manufacturers. Standard economic analysis of the welfare effects of price discounting concludes that consumers benefit when total sales volume increases, which is plausible in the case of pharmaceuticals. More generally, the managed care revolution depends on the ability of health-care plans to negotiate discounted rates in return for shifting market share to network providers and suppliers, thereby increasing their volume. Selective contracting in return for price discounts is fundamental to controlling costs for hospital and physician services, as well as for pharmaceuticals.

Second, in the case of pharmaceuticals that incur significant costs of research and development, charging different prices to different markets or countries is consistent with the most appropriate feasible (second-best optimal) method of paying for R&D costs. R&D is a global joint cost that serves all consumers, in all countries of the world that use the product. This R&D expense cannot be attributed to any single group rather than another. There is no presumption that the best way to recoup this cost is for all consumers to pay equally. On the contrary, the theory of Ramsey pricing (Ramsey 1927) concludes that in such contexts, charging different prices to different consumers based on demand elasticity is the most efficient way of covering the joint costs. The application of these principles to price differentials within the United States and between different countries is discussed in detail in Danzon (1998).

Discounting Does Not Imply Cost-Shifting

The Minority Staff Reports argue that discounting to some customers leads to higher prices for other customers. The source cited for this is a Standard and Poor's Report.[19] But this argument is inconsistent with rational self-interested behavior on the part of a firm. Simple economic theory shows that if a firm serves two separate customer groups, say A and B, which differ in their price sensitivity, that firm would maximize its net revenue by charging different prices in the two markets. It would charge a higher price in the market that is less price-sensitive, say market A, other things being equal. If demand in market B now becomes more price-sensitive, the firm will lower its price in that market. But the price to the less price-sensitive market A is unaffected—indeed, to raise the price to group A would actually reduce net revenue, since by assumption it had already set the price to maximize net revenue in that market. By analogy, increased price-sensitivity in the managed care market has led suppliers to offer discounts in that market, but this does not affect prices to other customers, as long as the markets are independent.

If the manufacturer is required to charge the same price in both markets, then the single price will be within the range of prices that would have been charged, had markets been independent. The evidence from GAO (1994b) and CBO (1996) confirms that for similar reasons, the OBRA 1990 requirement that manufacturers give a best price discount to Medicaid equal to the largest discount given to any other private purchaser led to a reduction in discounts available to HMOs and other private purchasers (see table 3–1 and figure 3–2).

6
Policy Implications

Appropriate pharmaceutical coverage for the elderly is an important policy issue. Roughly two-thirds of seniors do have coverage, either through employer-sponsored or individually purchased Medigap coverage; through Medicaid, which covers out-of-pocket expense for seniors with low incomes; or by choosing an HMO that offers drug benefits, under the Medicare + Choice program. A recent study (Davis 1999) reports that 35 percent of seniors do not have outpatient drug coverage.

A full analysis of the issue of appropriate outpatient drug coverage for seniors is beyond the scope of this study. If coverage is provided, however, the evidence here and from other sources makes clear that this should not be simply indemnity coverage, which would make demand in this market segment even more inelastic and would increase costs. A preferred approach is to give seniors the choice between competing private-sector health plans that offer a managed pharmacy benefit, as in many Medicare + Choice options or the Federal Employee Health Benefits Program. Compared with traditional indemnity coverage, a managed pharmacy benefit would yield savings not only from discounts on manufacturer prices but also savings on retail distribution markups and use of mail order, in addition to quality control. As noted above, the GAO (1997a) found that, of the savings to the Federal Employee Health Benefit Program from use of a pharmacy benefit manager (PBM), roughly 50 percent resulted from discounts achieved on distribution costs.

There have been proposals that would extend to the Health Care Financing Administration (HCFA) the ability to contract directly with PBMs or to use other, private-sector best commercial practices to provide prescription drugs to Medicare beneficiaries as an add-on to traditional Medicare. Although this extension might seem logical, managed pharmacy benefits are more appropriately provided as part of an integrated benefit, as in many private-sector health plans. If a pharmacy benefit is simply added to traditional Medicare, it is likely to become one component of traditional Medicare's current silo-budgeting approach to cost control. Each service component—hospitals, physicians, home health, pharmacy, and so forth—would likely be subject to separate budget controls, implemented by fee or price controls, which provide no incentive for providers to seek efficient integration and mixture of medical services.

Another alternative, which has been proposed in HR 664, is to require sales to the retail segment at Federal Supply Schedule prices. By increasing the volume of business at FSS prices but without increasing price responsiveness, this proposed approach is likely to result in higher prices to private managed care and to government customers who currently receive discounts, as occurred after enactment of the Medicaid best price provision. Note that this prediction is entirely consistent with the analysis detailed at the end of chapter 5. There it was argued, based on economic theory, that as long as the two market segments—the relatively price-inelastic retail sector and more price-elastic managed care/group purchasing organization (GPO) sector—are separate, the prices in the two markets are set separately. Therefore, giving a discount to the managed care/GPO sector does not result in a price increase in the retail sector. By contrast, once the retail sector is required to get the same price as the FSS, which is already required to get at least the best price given to the managed care/GPO sector, the two markets are no longer separate. A price discount given to the managed care/GPO sector must be matched in the retail sector. A manufacturer would now rationally charge a price based on the weighted average price elasticity in the two sectors. This will be above the previous price to the managed care/GPO sector. Hence, tying the retail sector to the FSS price will result in an increase in prices to managed care/GPO and federal and nonfederal purchasers. This effect is likely to be large, because of the relatively large size of the price-inelastic retail sector.

The effect of requiring manufacturers to charge the same price in all market segments was illustrated following the enactment of the Omnibus Budget Reconciliation Act (OBRA) (1990), as discussed above. This law tried to reduce Medicaid's prescription drug costs by requiring that manufacturers give state Medicaid programs rebates based on the best price given to other purchasers. Between 1991 and 1993, the median best price discount given to HMOs declined from 24.4 percent to 14.2 percent; for GPOs the median best price discount declined from 27.8 percent to 15.3 percent (GAO 1994b). Thus, by the first quarter of 1993, the median best price discount to private managed purchasers had fallen to about the minimum 15 percent rebate required by OBRA, as predicted by simple economics (figure 3–1).

Similarly, the losers from a requirement that retail customers be offered FSS prices would be managed care and other federal and nonfederal customers, who would face increased prices. The restrictions on discounts could also reduce best price rebates to Medicaid and hence increase taxpayer costs of financing the Medicaid program. Pharmaceutical manufacturers would also lose in the short run, from the loss of flexibility to adapt to the more complex market conditions that include managed and unmanaged customers. In the long run this would adversely affect incentives for investment in innovative products.

Moreover, there is no guarantee that any price decrease to pharmacists would be passed on to retail customers. Since demand in the unmanaged retail market is determined largely by physicians, who typically are unaware of prices charged by retail pharmacists, competition puts little pressure on pharmacists to pass on reductions in acquisition prices to the unmanaged, cash-paying patients. Consistent with this, pharmacists' margins are often higher for generic drugs than for branded drugs, because they do not fully pass through the lower acquisition cost of generics. Thus, a requirement that retail customers be offered FSS prices would result in a loss to managed care and GPO patients that would almost certainly exceed any gain from lower prices to unmanaged, retail customers.

Notes

1. *Prescription Drug Pricing in the United States: Drug Companies Profit at the Expense of Older Americans.* Minority Staff Report, Committee on Government Reform and Oversight, U.S. House of Representatives, September 25, 1998.

2. *Prescription Drug Pricing in the 1st Congressional District in Maine: An International Price Comparison.* Prepared for Rep. Thomas A. Allen, Minority Staff Report, Committee on Government Reform and Oversight, U.S. House of Representatives, October 24, 1998.

3. See, for example, Diewert (1987) and references therein.

4. The U.S. figure is from Intercontinental Medical Statistics (IMS) America. In particular, generic market share is negligibly small in countries with strict price regulation for branded products, such as France and Italy.

5. The volume weight corresponds to the measure of price. For example, if the price measure is price per gram, the weight is the number of grams; if the price is price per dose, the weight is the number of doses sold.

6. The FSS prices are apparently reported net of a mandatory 0.5 percent Industrial Funding Fee that "reimburses the VA for the costs of operating the Federal Supply Schedules Programs and recoups its operating costs from ordering activities" (U.S. Code Section 552.238.77).

7. The average manufacturer price (AMP) is typically about 2 percent below the manufacturer's list price, because of discounts routinely given to wholesalers.

8. For most of these products with FSS above FCP (72 per-

cent) the differential was less than 1 percent, and probably a consequence of the fee for the VA's administration of the FSS (GAO 1997b, p. 15 and footnote 17).

9. These products with an FSS price less than the FCP were on average 52 percent below the NFAMP, as of September 30, 1996 (GAO 1997, note 17).

10. The median is the midpoint of a distribution, such that half the observations fall below and half above that point.

11. These figures are for the Blue Cross-Blue Shield Plan. The other two plans in the study reported even smaller shares of savings attributable to manufacturer discounts and larger shares attributable to retail and mail-order pharmacy discounts.

12. The GAO (1997b) reports FSS sales at 1.5 percent of total pharmaceutical sales in the United States, citing data from the Intercontinental Medical Statistics (IMS).

13. *Prescription Drug Pricing Report: Minnesota's 6th Congressional District.* Minority Staff Report, Committee on Government Reform, U.S. House of Representatives, April 5, 1999.

14. GAO (1992) reported the average price for the market basket in the United States compared with its average price in Canada. It also reported the median of the price ratios.

15. These comparisons are based on IMS data for single-molecule drugs. The product is defined by molecule and 4-digit anatomical therapeutic category (MOL/ATC), regardless of manufacturer or brand name. The price for a multisource molecule is the weighted average price over all manufacturers of that compound for a particular 4-digit therapeutic category. The indexes compare price per IMS standard unit, averaging over all packs, strengths, and dosage forms of products in the molecule. The IMS standard unit is one tablet, one capsule, 10ml. of a liquid, and so forth, and is a rough proxy for a dose. This avoids bias that occurs if comparison is limited to a single pack. For more detail, see Danzon (1996) and Danzon and Kim (1998).

16. The PBM is an intermediary that negotiates and manages the drug benefit, in return for a fee. In many cases the PBM does not directly buy drugs.

17. For details of managed pharmacy benefit programs, see Novartis (1998).

18. Nobel laureate George Stigler first suggested this "survivor" test for relative efficiency. In any competitive market, firms whose product or service offers consumers greater value for money will tend to expand their market share, at the expense of firms whose products offer consumers a less desirable trade-off between cost, quality, and convenience.

19. Herman Saftlas, *Health Care: Pharmaceuticals, Industry Surveys 19-20*. Standard and Poor's, December 18, 1997.

References

AARP Public Policy Institute and the Lewin Group. 1997. "Out of Pocket Health Spending by Medicare Beneficiaries Age 65 and Older: 1997 Projections."

Anderson, G., and J. P. Poulier. 1999. "Health Spending, Access, and Outcomes: Trends in Industrialized Countries." *Health Affairs* 18: 178.

Berndt, Ernst R. 1994. "Uniform Pharmaceutical Pricing: An Economic Analysis." Washington, D.C.: AEI Press.

Berndt, Ernst R., Zvi Griliches, and Joshua G. Rosett. 1993. "Auditing the Producer Price Index: Micro Evidence from Prescription Pharmaceutical Preparations." *Journal of Business and Economic Statistics* 11.

Danzon, Patricia M. 1998. "Welfare Effects of Price Differentials for Pharmaceuticals in the U.S. and the EU." *International Journal of the Economics of Business*.

———. 1996. "The Uses and Abuses of International Price Comparisons." In *Competitive Strategies in the Pharmaceutical Industry,* ed. Robert Helms. Washington, D.C.: AEI Press.

Danzon, Patricia M., and Jeong D. Kim. 1998. "International Price Comparisons for Pharmaceuticals: Measurement and Policy Issues." *PharmacoEconomics*.

Davis, M., J. Poisal, G. Chulis, C. Zarabozo, and B. Cooper. 1999. "Prescription Drug Coverage, Utilization and Spending among Medicaid Beneficiaries." *Health Affairs*, January/February.

Diewert, W. E. 1987. "Index Numbers." In *The New Palgrave Dictionary of Economics*, ed. J. Eatwell, M. Milgate, and P. Newman. New York: Macmillan.

Emron. 1998. Managed Care Pharmacy Director CUE Program.

Griliches, Z., and I. Cockburn. 1996. "Generics and New Goods in Pharmaceutical Price Indexes." In *Competitive Strategies in the Pharmaceutical Industry,* ed. Robert Helms. Washington, D.C.: AEI Press.

Kongstvedt, Peter R. 1996. *The Managed Health Care Handbook,* third ed. Gaithersburg, Md.: Aspen.

Manning, R. 1997. "Products Liability and Prescription Drug Prices in Canada and the United States." *Journal of Law and Economics* 40.

Minority Staff Domestic Report. 1998a. Committee on Government Reform and Oversight, U.S. House of Representatives. *Prescription Drug Pricing in the United States: Drug Companies Profit at the Expense of Older Americans.* September 25.

Minority Staff International Report. 1998b. Committee on Government Reform and Oversight, U.S. House of Representatives. *Prescription Drug Pricing in the 1st Congressional District in Maine: An International Price Comparison.* October 24.

Minority Staff Report. 1999. Committee on Government Reform and Oversight, U.S. House of Representatives. *Prescription Drug Pricing Report: Minnesota's 6th Congressional District.* April 5.

NERA (National Economic Research Associates). 1998. *The Health Care System in Mexico.* London: Pharmaceutical Partners for Better Health Care.

Novartis. 1998. *Pharmacy Benefit Report: Trends and Forecasts.*

Ramsey, F. 1927. "A Contribution to the Theory of Taxation." *Economic Journal* 37: 47–61.

Saftlas, Herman. 1997. *Health Care: Pharmaceuticals, Industry Surveys 19–20*. Standard and Poor's. December 18.

Salomon Smith Barney. 1998. *The Search for Value in Global Pharmaceuticals.*

Sherer, F. 1997. "How U.S. Antitrust Legislation Can Go Astray: The Brand Name Prescription Drug Litigation." *International Journal of the Economics of Business* 4: 239–56.

U.S. Congressional Budget Office. 1996. "How the Medicaid Rebate on Prescription Drugs Affects Pricing in the Pharmaceutical Industry." January 1996.

U.S. General Accounting Office. 1992. "Prescription Drugs: Companies Typically Charge More in the United States than in Canada." GAO-HRD-92-110. Washington, D.C.

———. 1994a. "Prescription Drugs: Companies Typically Charge More in the United States than in the United Kingdom. GAO/HEHS-94-29. Washington, D.C.

———. 1994b. "Medicaid: Changes in Best Price for Outpatient Drugs Purchased by HMOs and Hospitals." GAO/HEHS-94-194FS. Washington, D.C.

———. 1997a. "Pharmacy Benefit Managers: FEHBP Plans Satisfied with Savings and Services, but Retail Pharmacies Have Concerns." GAO/HEHS-97-47. Washington, D.C.

———. 1997b. "Drug Prices: Effects of Opening Federal Supply Schedule for Pharmaceuticals Are Uncertain." GAO/HEHS-97-60. Washington, D.C.

U.S. Medicine, Inc. 1998. *Federal Market Facts.*

About the Author

PATRICIA M. DANZON is the Celia Moh Professor of Health Care Systems and Insurance at the Wharton School, University of Pennsylvania. She has held positions at the University of Chicago, Duke University, and the RAND Corporation.

The author is a fellow of the Institute of Medicine and of the National Academy of Social Insurance. She has been a consultant on international health care issues to the World Bank, the New Zealand government, the Asian Development Bank, and the U.S. Agency for International Development.

Ms. Danzon is an adjunct scholar of the American Enterprise Institute. She is the author of *Pharmaceutical Price Regulations: National Policies versus Global Interests* (AEI Press, 1997).

www.ingramcontent.com/pod-product-compliance
Lightning Source LLC
Jackson TN
JSHW011943131224
75386JS00041B/1531

* 9 7 8 0 8 4 4 7 7 1 3 3 5 *